Lupus and You

A Practical Guide to Understanding, Managing, and Living with Systemic Lupus Erythematosus

Compliments From
N.E. In Lupus Chapter
5401 Keystone Dr. Suite 202
Fort Wayne, IN 46825
219-482-8205

By Eric S. Schned, MD

Rheumatology Treatment & Resource Center
and Park Nicollet Clinic

HealthSystem Minnesota

Foreword

This book is intended to help people with systemic lupus erythematosus (SLE or lupus) and their families understand what lupus is, what effects it might have on their lives, and what they can do to help themselves and their doctors manage the disease. It is intended to be useful for persons newly diagnosed with lupus, but will also be of interest to those who have had lupus for some time or might wish to review material and learn about new advances in the treatment of the disease. It is not intended to replace your doctor. Each case of lupus is special and may be quite different from another person's disease. Only your doctor can answer specific questions about your personal medical situation.

This is the third edition of a publication originally written in 1972. A second edition was published in 1986, but a good deal of new information about lupus has occurred since then. I have endeavored to update and add new information to this version. The original booklets were lauded by many patients for their simplicity and clarity. As information about lupus has expanded, this booklet is somewhat longer than the previous two, but I hope I have kept it relatively clear and easy to understand. I have also retained the previous versions' emphasis on the patient's and family's roles as partners in the management of lupus.

This book is not intended to replace your doctor. Each case of lupus is special; only your doctor can answer specific questions about your personal medical situation.

John E. Schwarz, currently a board member of the Minnesota Chapter of the Lupus Foundation of America, originally perceived the need for a booklet on lupus and funded development of the first edition. He deserves special recognition and thanks for those efforts.

Doctor Donnell Etzweiler, emeritus president of the International Diabetes Center, Park Nicollet Medical Foundation, was instrumental in writing and producing the first edition of the booklet. His many contributions to patient education over a long career are widely known and greatly appreciated.

Doctor James L. Reinertsen, M.D., presently chief executive officer of HealthSystem Minnesota, the parent organization of Park

Nicollet Clinic, wrote the second edition of the book. The excellence of this writing is apparent from the enduring popularity of this booklet which annually has sold 3,000-4,000 copies. I owe him a great debt of thanks for many years of mentoring, sage advice and trusted friendship. He has been an inspiration to me in my work in rheumatology over the last 15 years, as he has been to many other doctors and health care professionals in many fields in our community.

I wish to thank my rheumatology colleagues at Park Nicollet Clinic — Doctors Scott Glickstein, John Schousboe, and Robert Tierney — for their medical advice and editing of the text and content of the book. I thank Raymond Bechtle, who has volunteered many hours of service to the Rheumatology Treatment & Resource Center at Park Nicollet, for his helpful and insightful comments. Janet Lima, manager of the Rheumatology Treatment & Resource Center, and Lois Amundson, administrative secretary, have provided expert review, support, and editing and typing skills, and I thank them for this. I also gratefully acknowledge the financial and moral support of the Institute for Research and Education, HealthSystem Minnesota, (Executive Vice President James Toscano) in developing this book. I am also deeply indebted to the Schott Foundation for ongoing support of the Rheumatology Treatment & Resource Center. This support has helped make the revision of this publication possible.

Finally, I owe a debt of gratitude to and express my love for my wife, Nancy, and my children, Molly, Daniel and Alex, for their forbearance, love and support in this and many other professional endeavors.

Eric S. Schned, MD
May 1997

Table of Contents

L upus erythematosus is a complex illness. It may cause many different symptoms and it may vary greatly from person to person. It may be confused with other diseases and it may take a long time to diagnose. People who are diagnosed as having lupus often have many questions about the disease. Some common questions will be addressed in the first section of this booklet. Many questions that are specific to your own condition are best answered by your doctor, who knows you best.

You will notice that some of the words in this book have been underlined. These key concepts and terms are defined in the glossary on pages 45-49.

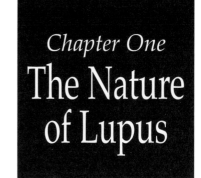

Chapter One
The Nature of Lupus

Lupus: An Introduction

What is lupus?

Lupus erythematosus is a chronic inflammatory disease that may affect many organs of the body. Let's break the description down into parts. Lupus is *chronic*. This means that although the course of the disease may fluctuate, with flare-ups and remissions, it usually lasts a lifetime. Lupus is *inflammatory*. This means that affected parts of the body may become red and swollen and painful. Pain, redness and swelling are signs of inflammation and are usually due to the body's normal reaction to foreign substances. A common example of inflammation is a sore throat (pharyngitis), when bacteria or a virus causes the throat to be sore, red, irritated and painful. In lupus, similar inflammation occurs in certain tissues and organs.

Lupus inflammation may affect many of the body's organs. The skin, joints, heart, lungs, nervous system — almost any part of the body — may become inflamed. Fortunately, lupus rarely affects all organs at the same time. In addition, many people have only one or a few organs that are ever affected. Because inflammation of the joints and muscles may cause aching and stiffness, lupus is sometimes called a rheumatic disease. It is *not* infectious, contagious, cancerous or malignant.

A recent survey suggests that almost two million Americans may have lupus.

How common is lupus?

Lupus is relatively common. A recent survey suggests that almost two million Americans may have lupus. It is more common than multiple sclerosis, leukemia, muscular dystrophy, cystic fibrosis and AIDS combined. It is much more common in women than in men and somewhat more common in Asians and African Americans than in white populations.

What does "lupus erythematosus" mean?

In Latin, "lupus" means "wolf" and "erythematosus" means "redness." Doctors described this disease a century or more ago. It seems that the skin rashes on the face of some people with lupus reminded doctors of a wolf face.

The Cause of Lupus

What causes lupus?

We know that lupus seems to be due to abnormalities in the body's immune system, but we don't know yet why these abnormalities occur. Normally, the immune system uses its powerful protectors — mainly protective proteins called antibodies and white blood cells (especially lymphocytes, neutrophils, and macrophages) — to fight off foreign substances, such as viruses, bacteria, and harmful chemicals, toxins and other substances.

In persons with lupus, however, an abnormality in the immune system causes the immune system to become "overactive." New antibodies and abnormal lymphocytes seem to lose the ability to distinguish between the body's own tissues and foreign substances. This unfortunate "confusion" means that some of the new antibodies and lymphocytes attack the body's own healthy tissues and cells. Therefore, doctors think of lupus as an "autoimmune" disease ("auto" means "self"). The immune system turns on the body itself.

Although there are quite a few ways in which autoimmunity can cause inflammation in lupus, two of the most common are shown in Figures 1 and 2. In Figure 1, specific "autoantibodies" (antibodies that are directed against a specific cell or tissue of the body) attack cells to cause damage

(continued on page 6)

Figure 1. Autoantibodies

In the diagram on the right, an antibody may attach to targets, called antigens, on cells or pieces of protein. Once the antibody attaches, a series of chemical reactions may lead to damage or destruction of the target cell.

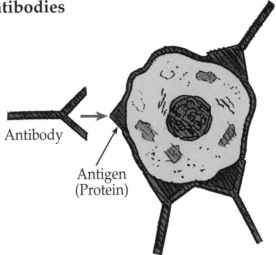

Antibody

Antigen (Protein)

Figure 2. Immune complexes

Sometimes, a foreign protein (AG) circulating freely in the bloodstream may be recognized by an antibody (AB) that binds to the protein. The foreign protein-antibody combination is called an "immune complex" (IC).

Blood Vessel Wall

Cross-Sectional Views of Blood Vessel

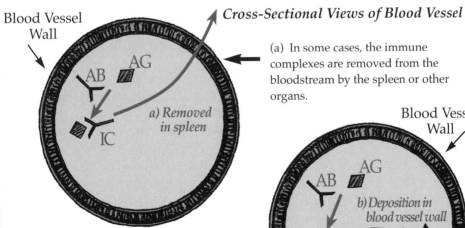

a) Removed in spleen

(a) In some cases, the immune complexes are removed from the bloodstream by the spleen or other organs.

Blood Vessel Wall

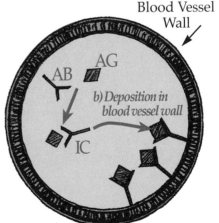

b) Deposition in blood vessel wall

(b) In other cases, the "immune complexes" may deposit in the walls of the blood vessels. This may lead to inflammation, swelling, obstruction of blood flow and injury or damage to nearby tissues.

(continued from page 4)

or inflammation. For example, specific antibodies that form against red blood cells can cause a type of anemia.

In Figure 2, other specific antibodies attach to certain proteins or particles ("<u>antigens</u>") to form "<u>immune complexes</u>." In many cases, these immune complexes circulate in the bloodstream and then may deposit in the walls of blood vessels. These deposits lead to local inflammation in the tissue and can cause damage to an organ or other problems. In some ways they resemble rust forming on pipes in your plumbing, leading to corrosion and leaks. Immune complexes are known to cause inflammation in the kidneys, skin, joints and other tissues.

Why do some people get lupus?

We don't know exactly why some persons are more likely to get lupus, but we do have some clues.

> *Women are much more likely to have lupus than men; almost 90 percent of people who have lupus are women.*

First, female hormones seem to play a role. Women are much more likely to have lupus than men; almost 90 percent of people who have lupus are women. Lupus develops most commonly during the years that women menstruate (from 12 to 50 years of age) — a time when female hormone levels are highest.

Some animals have diseases that resemble human lupus. In several strains of mice, females are highly susceptible to the disease. When these female mice are castrated, the disease is less severe. When male mice of the same strains are castrated or given female hormones, they develop lupus at high rates.

Second, heredity appears to *influence* whether a person gets lupus. For example, lupus is more common in African Americans and Asians than in whites. Certain genes that influence the function of the immune system are more common in people with lupus than in those without.

However, heredity alone does not cause lupus. Studies of identical twins, who have virtually identical genes, show that if one twin has lupus, the other has about a 50/50 chance of getting the disease. This frequency is much higher than in other people, but the fact that some twins don't get the disease means something else must be present or must happen to trigger the onset of lupus.

What triggers lupus?

Presumably, some event that occurs at just the right time in a person who is genetically predisposed to lupus might trigger the disease. It commonly occurs after viral infections, intense psychological stress and overexposure to sunlight. Other suspected triggers are some medications, chemicals, vaccinations and perhaps certain foods, such as alfalfa.

How serious is lupus?

Years ago, before doctors knew a lot about lupus, most cases that they diagnosed were quite serious. At that time, lupus was considered life-threatening.

Today, better tests and more awareness of the disease have allowed doctors to identify many more cases, most of which are quite mild. We know that there is a broad spectrum of severity of lupus, from the mild (common) to the very serious (uncommon). Moreover, because of today's improved treatments, many problems that were previously considered serious can now be managed successfully. Lupus must be taken seriously, but the outlook for most people with lupus is quite favorable.

You should discuss with your physician the seriousness of your condition. Proper care and early treatment can keep mild problems with lupus from becoming serious.

Description of the Disease

What are the "types" of lupus?

There are several "types" of lupus. Systemic lupus erythematosus, sometimes abbreviated "SLE," is the most common form and may affect almost any organ of the body. The symptoms that a person has depend on the organs affected, and the severity of the disease depends on the extent of organ inflammation or injury. The next section describes some of the common symptoms and problems associated with lupus.

Discoid lupus is a less common form of lupus. It involves only the skin, usually affecting the face, scalp, ears, or upper arms. The skin in these areas may become firm, tender, red, and scaly, and scarring may occur. Discoid lupus is more common in African American people.

"Drug-induced" lupus is sometimes considered a third type of lupus. It is different from the other two types, and medical scientists don't quite know how to classify it. Drug-induced lupus is caused by certain medications. Some of the most commonly implicated medications are those that are used to treat abnormal heart rhythms, high blood pressure, epileptic seizures, infections and other conditions. Procainamide, hydralazine, phenytoin and isoniazid are examples. A few weeks or months after people take these medicines, symptoms that resemble lupus may develop, and abnormal antibodies resembling those in lupus may appear. When the medications are stopped, the symptoms and abnormal blood tests will eventually disappear.

It should also be noted that quite a few people may develop diseases that resemble lupus but don't quite "fit" the typical case. Some may have symptoms that "overlap" with diseases that are considered "cousins" of lupus, such as rheumatoid arthritis or a muscle disease called polymyositis. Doctors recognize that these people don't quite have lupus and may refer to the disease as "overlap" connective tissue disease or "lupus-like" disease.

Most of the information in this booklet is useful for all three types of lupus. If you have questions about your type of lupus and the information included here, be sure to talk with your doctor.

What are the symptoms of lupus?

Lupus can cause many different symptoms. They may be quite different from person to person. Doctors often say that no two people with lupus have the exact same disease. While some people with lupus may have many symptoms, most people have just a few. Most people manage without making major changes in their lifestyles. Some of the most common symptoms are fatigue; widespread aching in the muscles, joints and chest; low-grade fevers (99.5° to 100.5° F); and depression. Many people with these symptoms say they feel like they have the "flu," but unlike the real flu, the symptoms never seem to go away. People with lupus may not know exactly what's wrong with them; they just know they don't feel good.

Lupus can be frustrating for patients and their families until they understand what's going on. Early on, lupus may be very difficult to diagnose. Its most common symptoms occur in many other illnesses and are often vague and difficult to describe. Often, patients think that others do not understand or believe them because they look good but feel lousy. Doctors, family and friends may think the person with lupus is exaggerating or faking.

The following symptoms and signs are common in lupus. Those that are considered most specific for lupus are marked with an asterisk and shown in Table 1.

Joint pain, swelling, and stiffness*, similar to that in <u>arthritis</u>. Usually, aching occurs in many joints, especially hands, wrists, shoulders, knees, ankles, and feet. Fortunately, lupus arthritis seldom damages the joints severely.

"Pleuritic" chest pain*. Pleuritic pain means that it hurts to breathe in and out. It is usually due to inflammation of the outer lining of the lungs (pleuritis*) or the sac surrounding the heart (<u>pericarditis</u>*).

Skin rashes. Lupus skin rashes can vary. The classic "butterfly rash"* is a bright red rash that may be scaly and may itch or burn and spreads over the bridge of the nose and the cheeks. It looks like a butterfly. Other rashes can occur on the upper chest, neck, back, arms, hands, or scalp. They are usually red and scaly.

Occasionally, people with systemic lupus may have discoid rashes*, which may scar. These rashes are frequently raised and red and may have pits or depressed areas in them. Sometimes they cause increased skin pigmentation.

Exposure to sun may cause lupus rashes to appear or to worsen. This is called <u>photosensitivity</u>.*

<u>Alopecia</u>*. Some people may develop patchy areas of hair loss, called alopecia.

Dry eyes and dry mouth*. This condition is called <u>Sjogren's syndrome</u> and is due to inflammation of the tear glands and the salivary glands.

Table 1. Lupus Symptoms and Signs

The following symptoms and signs are considered most specific for lupus:

- *Joint pain, swelling and stiffness*

- *"Pleuritic" chest pain*

- *Butterfly rash*

- *Discoid rash*

- *Photosensitivity*

- *Patchy areas of hair loss*

- *Dry eyes and dry mouth*

- *Kidney inflammation*

- *Low white blood cell count*

- *Low platelet count*

- *Blood clotting problems*

Raynaud's phenomenon. In cold weather, some people note changes in the color of their fingers or toes. They may turn pale-white at first and then become blue or purple or red.

Serious inflammation of certain organs. While somewhat less common, the following conditions can occur in lupus:

• *Kidney inflammation, called <u>glomerulonephritis</u>** or <u>nephritis</u>*, may not be associated with any symptoms at all, but may be discovered by finding red blood cells or protein in the urine. In some cases, nephritis may cause puffy swelling of the ankles, a change in the color or frequency of the urine, and high blood pressure.

• *The brain and nervous system* may sometimes be affected in lupus. Some symptoms of this are headaches, numbness or weakness on one side of the body, seizures, depression, mood swings, and difficulty with memory or concentrating.

Blood system abnormalities. The types of blood system abnormalities that may develop include the following:

• <u>*Anemia,*</u> or low red blood cell count, may cause lightheadedness, weakness, shortness of breath, or rapid heart beat.

• <u>*Leukopenia*</u>*, or low white blood cell count, may not cause problems, but if the count is too low it may lead to infections.

• <u>*Thrombocytopenia,*</u>* or low platelet count, can lead to bleeding or bruising since the platelet cells are important in blood clotting.

• *Clotting problems.* Small numbers of people with lupus may have certain autoantibodies in their blood that predispose them to forming clots in their veins or arteries. These antibodies are called <u>antiphospholipid antibodies</u>* (the two most common are called the <u>lupus anticoagulant</u> and <u>anticardiolipin antibodies</u>). Depending on where the clots form, a person may have a heart attack, a stroke, or phlebitis (which usually causes pain and swelling in the calf or thigh). Some women with antiphospholipid antibodies may have a higher rate of miscarriage (see "Can women with lupus have children?" on page 12).

Like any chronic illness, lupus may affect other bodily functions that are not directly related to the disease. For instance, menstrual periods may become irregular or stop. Decreased appetite, weight loss and disturbed sleep also occur.

Danger signs

Several symptoms may indicate that relatively serious problems are occurring or are about to occur. Call your doctor immediately (even at night or on the weekend) or get to a medical facility promptly if any of the following occur:

- Severe chest pain
- Severe shortness of breath, especially if sudden
- Chills or temperature over 101.5 degrees, especially if sudden
- Confusion
- Difficulty speaking or jumbled words
- Severe headache
- Fainting
- Seizures
- Severe cough, especially with sputum production, fever and/or shortness of breath
- Sudden swelling of the feet and ankles
- Weakness or numbness of arms or legs

Other, less serious signs — such as cold symptoms, fatigue, low-grade fever (under 100.5 degrees), skin rash and sore joints — usually do not

A Sample Log

Some people like to keep a graph or record of certain specific measures daily or at other intervals — such as daily maximum temperatures, hemoglobin levels, etc.

Danger sign	When it started	When it stopped
• Fever: 99.5 degrees	5/7/97	5/8/97
• Cold with head congestion	7/20/97	7/23/97
• Shoulder pain	8/15/97	8/20/97

require immediate attention. If any of these less serious symptoms occur, you should call your doctor's office or discuss them with your doctor at your next checkup.

Some people use a chart or a pocket planner to record their symptoms, temperature, medicines, and other information. A chart for your own use is in the section, "Preparing for your next exam" (page 37). An example of a personal chart appears in Chapter 4 (page 38). You may find using a chart helpful to keep track of symptoms that fluctuate — and to identify when certain problems arise.

Can women with lupus have children?

Many, probably most, women with lupus can and do have healthy children. However, because pregnancy can have serious consequences for the mother and the child, it should be carefully monitored with your doctor and experienced obstetricians and pediatricians. It is also important to have reliable support systems, including your spouse or partner, family and friends.

The following issues are important to people who are considering pregnancy:

Overall, there is a moderately increased risk of prematurity and miscarriage in women who have lupus. The *most favorable* time to get pregnant is when the disease is quiet or in remission and the mother is taking few or no medicines.

Women who have antiphospholipid antibodies (the lupus anticoagulant and/or anticardiolipin antibodies) have an increased risk of miscarriage. You should be tested for these antibodies as part of the preparation for pregnancy. Women who have kidney disease, brain inflammation or heart valve problems may also be at high risk for pregnancy-related complications. Despite these concerns, large numbers of women are able to conceive and complete successful pregnancies because of careful planning.

For the mother, there is always a chance that lupus may flare during pregnancy. Until recently it was thought that pregnancy increased the risk of lupus flares. However, recent studies suggest that the risk may not be much greater than for comparable women who are not pregnant.

As in all pregnancies, it is highly desirable to be on few or no medications at the time of conception or later in pregnancy. Many medications can be potentially harmful or damaging to the fetus. However, there are instances when women require treatment for medical problems that arise. You should always consult with your doctor or obstetrician before using any medications during pregnancy.

In general — and if possible — it is a good idea to be off medications for a few months prior to conception. This way, you and your doctor will be able to judge whether lupus is active or quiet and if it is a favorable time to get pregnant.

Some medications that women take for their lupus may harm the ovaries and make it difficult to become pregnant. One such drug is cyclophosphamide (Cytoxan), which may be used for kidney or brain inflammation.

Although most babies born to mothers with lupus are healthy, there are a few complications that the baby may have. A few babies may have a temporary rash on their faces or bodies for a few weeks or months after they are born. Some of these babies may have a temporary reduction in the number of blood cells.

This condition is called neonatal lupus. It is caused by antibodies from the mother that cross the placenta to the baby. The antibodies may persist in the baby for a few weeks or a few months and then disappear. Fortunately, the rash also fades away without leaving scars, and the low blood count returns to normal.

Rarely, a baby may be born with a very slow heartbeat (called congenital heart block). Some of these babies need to be treated with a pacemaker. This condition occurs rarely in babies whose mothers carry a special antibody, called <u>anti-SSA antibody</u> (also sometimes call <u>anti-Ro antibody</u>). This antibody may cross the placenta and attach to tissue that controls the rhythm of the fetus's growing heart.

Once a woman with lupus is pregnant, she will need frequent check-ups by her doctors. Sometimes special tests and special treatments may be necessary. Your doctor will review this with you before pregnancy.

Once in a while, lupus may flare a few weeks or months after delivery. Your doctor will want to follow you closely after you have given birth.

Outcomes of Lupus

How long will lupus last?

Lupus is a chronic disease. There is no known cure, but in most cases, symptoms can be controlled. Although doctors and medications play an important part in managing the disease, the person with lupus plays an equally important role. You should think of yourself, your doctors, your family, and your friends as a team. By balancing the different areas of your life, maintaining a positive attitude and learning as much as possible about lupus, you can better manage the disease.

Many people with lupus who have symptoms will become symptom-free for months or years, only to have symptoms reappear. "Remission" — the period when symptoms disappear — may be brought on by medicines or can occur spontaneously. Even during periods when the disease is active, symptoms may fluctuate weekly and even daily.

The time when symptoms reappear is called a "flare." While the causes of flares are unknown, you can decrease the chances of a serious flare by avoiding overexposure to the sun, pacing your work and resting to keep from becoming overly tired, maintaining regular living habits, getting adequate sleep, seeing your doctor regularly, and taking your medications as prescribed.

How is lupus treated?

Fortunately, effective treatment is available to most people with lupus. With a proper balance between rest and activity and strong teamwork between the person with lupus and his or her doctor, family, and friends, most people can successfully manage lupus. Chapter Three, entitled "Managing Lupus," deals with this issue in detail.

What research is being done?

Extensive research is underway to determine the cause of lupus and to find a cure for the disease. Much of the research focuses on the immune system, particularly the genes and viruses that may cause this system to lose control. Other work is aimed at understanding how organs become inflamed and damaged. Still other research is looking for new treatments to regain control of the immune system. Much work needs to be done before we fully understand lupus, but the future holds promise for improving treatment methods and even preventing the disease.

How can family and friends help?

By being supportive and understanding, family and friends can help the person with lupus manage and cope with his or her disease more effectively. For example, at times, the person with lupus may be too tired to do much of anything. Relatives and friends should understand this and should try to help whenever possible. At the same time, the family should encourage the person with lupus to continue to lead his or her life in as usual a manner as possible and not to give in to the disease.

Family members can help by trying to:

- learn as much as they can about lupus (the Lupus Foundation of America offers patient orientation and other educational seminars, newsletters, pamphlets, and other services);
- go with the patient to the doctor's office when possible — and if the patient agrees;
- encourage the patient to take prescribed medications and to follow treatment carefully;
- be aware of what might trigger a flare and of the danger signs that show a flare is about to occur; and
- be a good sounding board when the person wants to talk or express feelings.

Which doctors take care of people with lupus?

Your primary care doctor, such as a family practitioner or <u>internist</u>, may know you best and may be the first doctor to diagnose your condition. Primary care doctors manage and follow many people with lupus. <u>Rheumatologists</u> are subspecialists who are experienced and specially trained in managing the problems brought on by lupus. At times, depending on your condition, you may need to see other doctors, such as a <u>dermatologist</u> (skin specialist), <u>nephrologist</u> (kidney specialist), <u>neurologist</u> (brain and nervous system specialist), or other specialist.

How do you and your doctor know that you have lupus? There are three primary pieces of information that doctors rely on to make a diagnosis of lupus: a medical history (what you tell him or her), a detailed physical examination (what the doctor sees when he or she examines you), and laboratory tests (what blood, urine, X-ray and other tests reveal).

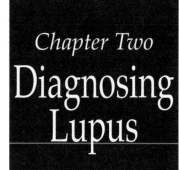

Chapter Two
Diagnosing Lupus

In some people, lupus is fairly easy to diagnose. These individuals usually have several "typical" or "classical" symptoms and signs that immediately cause the doctor to suspect lupus. The asterisked symptoms described on pages 9-10 make doctors think of lupus right away. In addition, people with lupus often have groups of symptoms that together point to lupus rather than other diseases.

A young woman with a "butterfly" facial rash, fever, joint pains, pleurisy, thinning hair, anemia, and urine containing protein would represent a very classical case of lupus; doctors would not think of much else.

On the other hand, quite frequently lupus may be very difficult to detect and diagnose. People may have symptoms that are vague and nonspecific, no clear-cut abnormalities on a physical exam, and minimal or no abnormalities on laboratory testing. What's more, the symptoms may fluctuate and be spread out over months or years. Remember, each case of lupus is different. Any number and combination of symptoms may be present, and any part of the body can be affected. When only one or two symptoms are present, they may not be enough for the doctor to be certain that lupus is the cause.

For example, a middle-aged woman with fatigue, aching in the muscles and joints, and anemia could have lupus, but she might also have early rheumatoid arthritis, hypothyroidism, cancer, a virus, Lyme disease, or quite a few other conditions.

In situations where it just isn't clear yet if lupus may be the cause of problems, it is wise for the physician and patient to agree that the diagnosis is uncertain at the time. Over time, certain new symptoms or new signs, such as a rash or abnormal blood tests, will develop. At that time, a definitive diagnosis of lupus can be made.

The Medical History

What your doctor will want to learn about

Your medical history provides vital information for the doctor. Of special importance is information about past occurrences of anemia, arthritis, skin rashes, sensitivity to the sun, dry eyes or dry mouth, unexplained fevers, hair thinning or hair loss, pleurisy, chronic fatigue, and a "false-positive test for syphilis" (see "Laboratory Testing" below). Sometimes the symptoms of lupus start years before it is diagnosed, and lupus may have been diagnosed as some other condition.

In addition, the doctor will want detailed information about your current and recent symptoms. Before you see the doctor, think about the way you have been feeling and note when each symptom began, how often each symptom occurred, how long each symptom lasted, and the severity of each symptom.

Your doctor will use past and present information that you provide, as well as past medical records, to begin to formulate ideas about what is going on with you and whether lupus might be a consideration.

The Physical Examination

What your doctor will look for

After taking a medical history, your doctor will give you a complete physical examination to gather more information. At your first visit and at some other visits, your doctor will pay special attention to your skin, hair, fingers and nails, mouth, joints, lymph glands, lungs and heart, liver, spleen, and neurologic system to detect signs of lupus.

Laboratory Testing

What tests your doctor may order

If your medical history and physical examination cause your doctor to suspect lupus, he or she will probably order laboratory tests. Some tests determine whether certain parts of your body, such as the blood cells, kidneys or liver, are affected or injured. Other tests are useful to diagnose or exclude lupus. It is very important to realize that no laboratory test is perfect; tests must be *interpreted* by the doctor. Usually, the tests *alone* do not permit the doctor to diagnose lupus. However, *in combination with the medical history and physical examination*, laboratory tests can confirm a diagnosis of lupus.

The following are the most common tests that doctors order when they are trying to diagnose lupus or to follow the progress of the disease:

- *Urinalysis*. This urine test reveals whether protein or red blood cells or white blood cells are present. If so, the kidneys may be inflamed.

- *Creatinine clearance*. This is a urine specimen that is collected over 24 hours. It is a very accurate way of determining how well the kidneys are working.

- *Twenty-four-hour urine protein collection*. This is a urine specimen that is collected over 24 hours. It is a very accurate way of determining exactly how much protein is leaking into the urine from inflamed or injured kidneys.

- *Tests on blood specimens*:

(1) *Complete blood count (CBC)*. This test measures the three main cells in the blood — red cells, white cells, and platelets — and can tell the doctor if the counts might be low from lupus or other causes.

(2) *Creatinine*. This test accurately measures how well the kidneys are working. The higher the value, the worse the kidneys are functioning.

(3) *Sedimentation rate ("sed rate")*. This is a rough measure of inflammation throughout the body. It may serve as a general guide in treatment.

(4) *C-reactive protein (CRP)*. This is an alternative test for inflammation.

(5) *Fluorescent antinuclear antibody (FANA) test.* This very important test may be the first laboratory clue that a person has lupus. It is useful especially as a screening test for lupus.

The FANA test detects antibodies in the blood that are "turned against" parts of the body's cells, namely the nuclei. These are true autoantibodies. Ninety-eight percent of people with lupus have a positive FANA test. Therefore, a negative FANA test is usually a strong indicator that a person doesn't have lupus.

However, a positive FANA test must be interpreted quite cautiously; it should only be used with other clinical information. It is *not very specific*. Many healthy people (especially older people), patients with other connective tissue diseases (for example, rheumatoid arthritis, Sjogren's syndrome, or scleroderma), persons with certain other medical diseases (such as thyroid or liver problems), and people on certain medications (including some blood pressure or heart medicines) may also test positive.

When a person has a positive FANA test, it usually prompts the doctor to do several other, more specific tests for lupus.

(6) *__Anti-DNA antibodies__*. These autoantibodies are extremely important in the diagnosis of lupus. Lupus is essentially the only disease that gives a positive result with this test.

It is important to note that only 30 to 50 percent of people with lupus test positively for anti-DNA antibodies. Therefore, while a positive anti-DNA antibody test almost definitely means you have lupus, you might have lupus and *not* have a positive anti-DNA antibody test.

In some cases, the amount of this antibody detected in the blood corresponds with how active lupus is.

Blood Tests

The following tests are performed on blood specimens to help diagnose lupus:

- *Complete blood count (CBC)*
- *Creatinine*
- *Sedimentation rate*
- *C-reactive protein (CRP)*
- *Fluorescent antinuclear antibody (FANA) test*
- *Anti-DNA antibodies*
- *Complement*
- *Anti-Smith antibodies*
- *Anti-SSA and anti-SSB antibodies*
- *Partial thromboplastin time (PTT)*
- *Anti-cardiolipin antibodies*

(7) *__Complement__ (C3, C4, CH50, and others)*. Complement refers to a group of proteins in the body that are important in defending the body against infections. These proteins are also often involved in inflammation in many parts of the body.

When lupus inflammation is severe, complement proteins may be used up. This is detected as decreases in the normal levels of these proteins. Low complement levels are frequently present when the kidneys are inflamed (glomerulonephritis).

(8) *Anti-Smith (Anti-Sm) antibodies*. These autoantibodies, like anti-DNA antibodies, are very specific for lupus, although they are present in only about one quarter of people with this disease.

(9) *Anti-SSA and anti-SSB antibodies*. These autoantibodies are found in most people with Sjogren's syndrome (see "What are the symptoms of lupus?" on page 8) and up to half of people with lupus. Some individuals with lupus who get rashes that are extremely sensitive to the sun often have anti-SSA antibodies. One out of 25 women with anti-SSA antibodies who are pregnant will have a baby with a very slow heartbeat, called congenital heart block (see page of 13 "Can women with lupus have children?").

(10) *Partial thromboplastin time (PTT)*. This test measures how well a part of the blood clotting system works. People who have a special antibody, called the lupus anticoagulant, will have a high or prolonged PTT. These people have an increased risk of clotting in their veins or arteries, and pregnant women with the lupus anticoagulant have a high risk for miscarriage. Treating such women with blood thinners may promote a successful pregnancy.

(11) *Anti-cardiolipin antibodies*. These antibodies are similar to the lupus anticoagulant. Their presence indicates that a person has an increased risk of developing blood clots in veins or arteries. Pregnant women have an increased risk of miscarriage.

• *Biopsy*. A biopsy is a procedure whereby a very small piece of living tissue is removed from an organ and then examined under a microscope or tested. Biopsies of the skin, kidneys, muscle, lung and rarely other tissues are often done to help determine whether it is lupus or another condition that is responsible for the inflammation or damage to a tissue.

• *MRI scan; CTT (CAT) scan*. These special techniques can "scan" or see tissues or parts of the body three-dimensionally. They are very valuable in determining (1) whether inflammation or damage may be present in such areas as the brain, chest, abdomen and spine, and (2) whether a problem in these areas might be due to lupus or some other condition.

Living with Uncertainty

What if the diagnosis is uncertain? Medicine is not a perfect science. Diagnosing lupus is sometimes quite easy and straightforward; on the other hand, it can be very difficult or uncertain despite careful evaluation and testing. The medical history, physical examination, and even laboratory tests may lead the doctor to *suspect* lupus, but a firm and definite diagnosis cannot be made.

Without more proof, the doctor will not want to say for certain that the person has or does not have SLE . This uncertainty or hesitancy is sometimes quite difficult for both the patient and the doctor to understand and accept.

What can be done when uncertainty about the diagnosis exists?

First, the doctor and the patient should talk about the inconclusiveness of the diagnosis. The patient should understand what *other* possibilities exist as well.

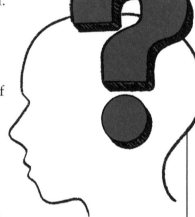

Second, the patient or the doctor might seek a second opinion from an expert in lupus care.

Third, the doctor can recommend close and careful observation over time, with repetition of tests in the future. In most individuals, if lupus is untreated, it will gradually progress over time so that the diagnosis becomes clear later and specific treatment may be begun.

In any instance, the patient deserves sympathy and understanding in dealing with uncertainty.

I t is a cardinal rule in treating lupus that, depending on what problems are occurring, the treatment for the disease will vary from one person to the next. Treatment will be different for rashes than for arthritis, and treatment for kidney inflammation will not be the same as for dry eyes. In addition, lupus may include periods of flares and remissions. Thus, treatment will typically change over time.

As a result, it's very important to follow your doctor's advice. You and your doctor need to be a "team" that communicates well and understands each other. Successful treatment of lupus usually starts with changes in a person's attitude, includes some changes in diet and activities and lifestyle, and almost always involves medications.

Let's look at these areas.

Your Attitude: Treating Yourself Well

A positive attitude will help in managing lupus. It is difficult not to worry or even to feel sad, angry or frustrated at times. In fact, to some degree this is natural. However, it is important to try to develop a positive attitude. There is growing evidence that positive attitudes can be beneficial in outcomes of lupus, whereas depression or anger might be harmful.

There is growing evidence that positive attitudes can be beneficial in outcomes of lupus, while depression or anger might be harmful.

There are some things you can work on to develop a positive attitude. Learn as much as possible about your disease. Ask your doctor about things that bother you. Talk about your problems with friends and family.

Sometimes it is difficult to find the right balance between sharing your worries and becoming worrisome to others. There are two extremes to avoid: keeping your worries completely to yourself or talking about lupus or your fears constantly. If you've never talked with anyone about your fears and concerns regarding lupus, try to do so. On the other hand, if lupus becomes your main topic of conversation, you may be letting it take over your life. Try to find the right balance. If you're having

Chapter Three
Managing Lupus

trouble dealing with some personal issues, talk to your doctor about getting professional help or join a support group.

Fortunately, most people with lupus can expect to lead full lives. They enjoy productive careers, recreational activities, marriage and children. Don't sell yourself short. Many people with lupus do not live up to their potential primarily because of their fears concerning the disease—not because of any major physical limitations. Don't let lupus become an excuse for other problems that are unrelated to your illness.

Sometimes you may follow your doctor's orders and take medicines as prescribed — and lupus flares may still occur. In other words, lupus doesn't always "follow the rules." It is important not to become discouraged or to feel guilty when this happens. This is when you need to stay in close touch with your doctor and your support systems.

General Lifestyle

Having lupus doesn't change your basic needs for healthy living: buckle your seatbelt, eat sensibly, get enough sleep, exercise regularly, and avoid tobacco and overuse of alcohol and other drugs.

Lupus may make some special demands on your lifestyle at times, especially during flares. Most people get pretty tired during flares because of the inflammation in their systems. During these periods, get plenty of rest; you should try to get at least eight hours of sleep a day, possibly more. A rest in the morning or a nap in the afternoon can be helpful. You may not need as much rest during remissions, but don't try to make up for lost time all at once. Don't overwork yourself. Reserve some energy.

Exercise

Exercise can be very valuable for people with lupus. Two types of exercise may be appropriate. Regular aerobic exercise is important for general health reasons — to keep weight down, to improve cardiorespiratory conditioning and stamina, and to improve cholesterol levels. If you have arthritis, you still want to do aerobic exercise, but you probably should limit it to low-impact activity (such as walking, biking, or swimming). You may want advice from a professional.

In addition, persons with arthritis will benefit from joint exercises — range of motion, stretching, and gradual strengthening exercises — to keep joints and soft tissues supple and strong. It is often advisable to get personalized instructions in joint exercise from a trained physical therapist.

Protection from the Sun

Twenty to twenty-five percent of people with SLE are sensitive to the sun. Exposure may cause skin rashes to develop or flare on the face, chest, arms and elsewhere. These may burn or itch, and occasionally they can scar. In some cases, highly sensitive people may get a generalized flare of their lupus with fatigue, joint pains, weakness, nausea, fevers, and kidney or lung inflammation. The sunlight may affect you even if it is cloudy, and you should watch out for sunlight that reflects off of water (if you are boating or at the beach), snow (if you are skiing) and even glass or mirrors.

For the most part, people with lupus should avoid direct and indirect sunlight, although limited exposure to the sun is usually safe for most people. Walking in the shade, going to ball games, and sitting under umbrellas or on porches are safe and fun. There are many other similar activities that are safe and enjoyable. Using common sense generally works well for most people.

The following are some suggestions for limiting sun exposure:

• *Schedule outdoor activities before 10 a.m. or after 4 p.m.* You will avoid the sun's most intense rays which occur during the midday.

• *Wear protective clothing* — such as a hat with a brim, long-sleeved blouse and skirt or slacks, long-sleeved dress, or long-sleeved shirt and pants. There are many types of special sun-protective clothing available through catalogs or stores.

• *Use sunscreen with a high sun protection factor (SPF).* For most people, an SPF of 15-20 is sufficient, but for highly sensitive individuals, sunscreen with an SPF of 40-50 or even higher may be necessary. There are many different sunscreens marketed; most contain para-aminobenzoic acid (PABA) or other agents that absorb ultraviolet (UV) light and prevent skin effects. Some sunscreens are creams and others are ointments. Some newer sunscreens are marketed as "chemical free." Some people are allergic to sunscreens. Talk with your pharmacist or dermatologist to learn about the sun protection for you.

- *Do not use tanning booths or beds.*

Some people wonder if light given off by TV sets or fluorescent lights or computer screens is dangerous. Usually this light has very small amounts of UV light and isn't a concern; however, in rare instances it can pose a problem. You should be alert if you notice rashes occurring with such exposures when you are at work, especially if the rashes are gone when you are not at work. Covers for fluorescent lights and special screens for computers are available.

Diet

There is very little scientific data to suggest that diet is beneficial or harmful in lupus, but some information indicates that alfalfa may aggravate lupus in animals. Thus, many doctors advise people with lupus to avoid alfalfa, even though there is no proof of problems with alfalfa in humans.

Many scientists are exploring whether certain vitamins, fish oils, antioxidants or food additives are helpful in decreasing inflammation in lupus, but it is too soon to make any recommendations.

You should follow principles of good nutrition:

- *Avoid obesity* by balancing your caloric intake.

- *Limit fat, particularly saturated fat, and cholesterol* (found in such foods as meats, dairy products, eggs, creams and rich desserts). Coronary artery disease may be somewhat more common in people with lupus. These dietary modifications can reduce this risk.

- *Add fiber to your diet* with whole-grain breads, cereals, vegetables and fruits, or commercial fiber agents.

- *Avoid salty foods and don't add table salt*, especially if you have kidney disease or hypertension.

- *Choose foods from all the major food groups*: breads, grains, and cereals; fruits and vegetables; fish, lean meat, poultry; dairy products.

- *Include foods and milk that contain adequate amounts of calcium* to prevent osteoporosis.

In some cases, special diets *are* necessary. If high blood pressure exists, most people should limit salt and increase calcium moderately. If you have kidney damage, your doctor may recommend a low-protein diet. Sometimes medications or kidney disease may affect cholesterol levels and you may need a special low-cholesterol and low-fat diet. Certain types of anemia may benefit from iron or vitamin supplements. Your doctor may suggest that you see a nutritionist or dietitian to help you plan these special diets.

Individuals with lupus often receive suggestions concerning fad or "miracle" diets; mega-vitamins; "natural," holistic, or herbal supplements; or "curative" therapies. Usually, there is no valid, scientific evidence to support the benefits of any of these products. Most so-called "evidence" comes from anecdotes or personal testimony that, unfortunately, can be very misleading. Indeed, in some cases, the "therapy" can be harmful and expensive. For example, high doses of Vitamin B_6 can cause severe nerve damage, and high doses of Vitamin A and Vitamin D can cause other problems. Information on diet and disease is constantly being updated. Ask your doctor for the latest information on foods and vitamins and other nutritional supplements.

Medical Therapy

As you can see, there is much more to treating and managing lupus than medications alone. However, medications are an important part of the lupus care plan. It is important to realize that there are no cures for lupus. However, a continually growing number of medications can ease symptoms and control modest flares, and other, more powerful ones can treat serious problems, such as kidney, brain and heart inflammations.

When your doctor prescribes any medication, you should learn as much as you can about it and carefully follow your doctor's advice. If you have questions about your medications, ask your doctor, pharmacist or nurse.

Remember: All medications, including over-the-counter products, "natural" treatments, herbs, vitamins and prescriptions, have *risks* as well as benefits. For any problem that you and your doctor want to treat, you always want to be certain that the potential benefits outweigh the possible risks.

How is lupus treated with medicines? Are all people treated with steroids? Treatment for lupus differs from one person to the next. It is tailored for the individual, and several types of medications are used. Each type serves a special function. For example, treatment of arthritis and rashes will call for different medications than treatment of kidney inflammation or anemia.

The following medications and treatments are commonly used in lupus care.

Aspirin

Use. These medications work by reducing inflammation caused by lupus in some parts of the body. They are commonly used to treat joint pains (arthralgia), arthritis, muscle aches (myalgias) and pleurisy. For many people with mild lupus, rest and aspirin may be the only treatment needed.

Preparations. There are quite a few different aspirin preparations available. In general, buffered and enteric-coated aspirins are preferred and are less irritating to the stomach.

Side effects. For the side effects of aspirin, please see pages 29-30.

Non-steroidal anti-inflammatory drugs (NSAIDs)

Use. In addition to aspirin, many other "non-steroidal anti-inflammatory drugs" or NSAIDs (pronounced "en-sedz") are available by prescription and over-the-counter. They are called "non-steroidal" because they are not steroids.

Preparations. By and large, NSAIDs are not dramatically different from aspirin, although many of them are quite a bit more expensive. For some people, however, NSAIDs do seem to work better than aspirin; they also may be better tolerated than aspirin. It is impossible to predict which NSAID might work, so it is a reasonable idea to start with one (perhaps a cheaper brand or a generic agent), try it, and then try two or three more in a row until you find one that works well. Table 1 (page 29) provides a list of commonly recommended NSAIDs.

In many instances, you might need your NSAID or aspirin only during flares. In general, however, NSAIDs work somewhat better when they are taken regularly as prescribed, rather than sporadically.

Table 1: Common NSAIDs

Generic Name	Brand Name
ibuprofen	Motrin, Advil, Nuprin, Rufen
sulindac	Clinoril
naproxen	Naprosyn, Aleve
naproxen sodium	Naprelan, Anaprox
indomethacin (immediate release)	Indocin (immediate release)
indomethacin (slow release)	Indocin SR 75
piroxicam	Feldene
flurbiprofen	Ansaid
ketoprofen	Orudis, Oruvail
diclofenac	Voltaren XR Voltaren
meclofenamate	Meclomen
fenoprofen	Nalfon
diflunisal	Dolobid
tolmetin	Tolectin
oxaprozin	Daypro
etodolac	Lodine
nabumetone	Relafen
acetylsalicylic acid (aspirin)	Ecotrin, Zorprin, many others
salsalate	Disalcid
choline magnesium salicylate	Trilisate

It is very important to take your medicine as prescribed. Too much medicine may cause serious side effects; too little may not relieve your symptoms properly. As a rule of thumb, you should not take aspirin with other NSAIDs, or two different NSAIDs at the same time, without your doctor's approval.

Side effects. Although reasonably safe, NSAIDs and aspirin do have several potentially serious side effects (see Table 2, page 30).

Stomach irritation. In some cases, NSAIDs can cause nausea, heartburn, abdominal pain and cramping. More seriously, they can lead to gastritis or stomach ulcers, which can cause severe pain, bleeding, or rarely, perforation. NSAIDs SHOULD ALWAYS BE TAKEN WITH FOOD. If you get stomach pains, consult your doctor promptly; he or she may recommend stopping the medications, using a different one, or taking antacids or other medicines to treat the stomach or to prevent ulcers.

Persons who have a history of ulcers or bleeding should never take aspirin or NSAIDs without consulting with their doctor first. Some medications (such as misoprostol) may be taken with the NSAID to prevent ulcers.

While you take aspirin or an NSAID, watch your stools. If they turn black, that may indicate serious stomach bleeding, and you should contact your doctor right away.

Kidney problems. Occasionally, NSAIDs or aspirin can cause some malfunction of the kidneys. This occurs most commonly in older people or in persons with underlying kidney disease, heart failure or other conditions. Your doctor may periodically check your blood or urine while you are taking NSAIDs to make sure your kidneys are OK.

Other effects. Sometimes people on NSAIDs or aspirin will experience other side effects, such as skin rash, fluid retention (ankle swelling), elevated blood pressure, minor bruising or easy bleeding.

Table 2: Side Effects of NSAIDs and Aspirin

√ *Stomach irritation*

√ *Kidney problems*

√ *Skin rashes*

√ *Fluid retention*

√ *Elevated blood pressure*

√ *Minor bruising*

√ *Easy bleeding*

Acetaminophen (Tylenol and other brand names)

Acetaminophen is an excellent moderate analgesic (pain killer) and antipyretic (fever reducer). There is no specific problem for which it is used to treat lupus, but it is very commonly used to relieve aches and pains, headaches and "flu" symptoms.

Steroids (cortisone-like medications)

Steroids (also called corticosteroids) are very powerful anti-inflammatory medications. They are related to cortisone, a critical hormone that is produced normally in the body by the adrenal glands. The dosages used during treatment of lupus (and many other diseases) often are much higher than the body produces naturally. Some commonly used steroids are Prednisone, Prednisolone, Dexamethasone and Triamcinolone.

Use. Steroids are generally used for more serious manifestations of lupus. In some cases, they can be life-saving, such as in treating brain inflammation, widespread blood vessel inflammation (vasculitis), or heart or lung disease. Steroids are commonly used in pill form or by injection in kidney inflammation (nephritis), muscle inflammation (myositis), severe arthritis, certain heart or lung inflammations, brain and neurological conditions, low platelets (thrombocytopenia), certain anemias (hemolytic anemia), severe skin rashes, and other situations. Creams or ointments are used for many skin rashes. Cortisone and lidocaine may be injected into inflamed or swollen joints.

Steroids are often used in high doses initially to control inflammation rapidly, and then the doses are lowered. Steroids have numerous potentially serious side effects, so the goal is to try to decrease the dose to the lowest level possible or to stop them.

AN IMPORTANT NOTE ABOUT STEROIDS

Never stop taking steroids abruptly. If you stop steroids abruptly, you can become very sick rapidly if the adrenals are "shut down." Weakness, vomiting and shock can occur. Never taper or stop steroids without clear advice from your doctor.

When people are on steroids for more than a week or two, the body becomes dependent on the drug. Stopping or tapering steroids should always be done gradually to allow the adrenal glands to start manufacturing cortisone again. The adrenal glands "shut down" when you take cortisone because they sense that there is more than enough cortisone in the body. When steroids are stopped, however, it can take the adrenal glands days, weeks, or even months before they "rev up" again to produce adequate amounts of cortisone.

Preparations. Steroids can be used in pill form, by injection into a muscle, intravenously, by injection into a joint, in eye drops, or in skin creams or ointments. The type used depends on the problem.

Side effects. Steroids are extremely effective medications, but, unfortunately, they carry significant risks. Not everyone will get serious side effects; some people are much more susceptible to certain side effects than others. Generally, the risks of getting side effects increase the longer you take them and the higher the doses over time. This is the reason doctors constantly try to taper the dose or sometimes add other drugs to get people off steroids or to lower doses.

The common side effects of steroids are described on the next page and summarized in Table 3.

Osteoporosis. Osteoporosis, or thinning of bones, may develop — sometimes rapidly — when people are on steroids for several months or years. Severe osteoporosis can cause fractures, especially in a hip or backbone. Post-menopausal women are at especially high risk for this since their bones start to thin at menopause.

Proper amounts of calcium, vitamin D, and exercise can lessen steroid-induced osteoporosis to some extent. Some new medicines appear to slow down or even partially reverse steroid-induced osteoporosis. You may be a candidate for one of these treatments and should check with your doctor about this. In some instances, it may be advisable to have a bone densitometry examination (a special X-ray-type test) to determine very precisely how dense your bones are.

Weight gain. This comes from a change in your metabolism while on steroids. Careful attention to diet, caloric intake and exercise can help prevent this.

Rounding of the face ("moon" face).

Acne.

Thinning of the skin. This condition can lead to easy bruising.

Stomach upset and irritation.

High blood pressure and fluid retention. People with high blood pressure may need to increase or add medication to control this.

High blood sugar, sometimes leading to diabetes. People who already have diabetes may have increased blood sugar levels and may need to make adjustments in their oral hypoglycemic medications and/or insulin.

Emotional changes or difficulty thinking properly. While on steroids, some people find themselves crying easily or getting depressed. Others don't sleep well.

Table 3: Possible Side Effects of Steroids

- √ Osteoporosis
- √ Weight gain
- √ Rounding of the face (moon face)
- √ Acne
- √ Thinning of the skin
- √ Stomach upset and irritation
- √ High blood pressure and fluid retention
- √ High blood sugar
- √ Emotional changes
- √ Bone collapse or osteonecrosis
- √ Infection

Bone collapse or osteonecrosis. This is rare. It usually occurs in hip bones and is associated with sharp pain when bearing weight.

Infection. In high doses, steroids depress the entire immune system, which can increase the risk of infections. You should notify your doctor if you observe symptoms or signs of a more serious infection than usual, such as green or yellow sputum, sinus discharge, cloudy and burning urine, infected skin wounds, ingrown toenails, or painful blisters on the face, chest, abdomen, back, arms or legs that might represent shingles (Herpes Zoster).

Antimalarial medications

Although no one knows exactly how they work, certain medications that are used to treat malaria also help control lupus. The most commonly used is hydroxychloroquine (Plaquenil).

Use. Antimalarial medications seem to work best for lupus skin rashes, arthritis and pleurisy. A recent research study showed that people who continued to take hydroxychloroquine for years had fewer and less severe flares of lupus than people who didn't. For this reason, your doctor may want you to take hydroxychloroquine for long periods of time.

Side effects. The antimalarial medications are relatively safe. Occasionally, they may cause a skin rash, stomach or intestinal upset, or loose stools.

Medications and Pregnancy

In general, a rule of thumb is that women should avoid medications as much as possible during pregnancy. Some medications are especially toxic to fetuses and can cause birth defects or intrauterine deaths. For example, cyclophosphamide, azathioprine, and methotrexate should be avoided in all but extreme circumstances.

Of course there are some instances when lupus must be treated during pregnancy. In those cases, your doctor will guide you towards acceptable treatments. For example, acetaminophen, aspirin, and ibuprofen may be reasonable choices for some people. Interestingly, steroids, even with their numerous side effects, do not cross the placenta in significant amounts and are, therefore, relatively safe for the fetus when the mother needs to take them.

Rarely they can cause problems in the retina of the eye; anyone taking antimalarial medications should visit an <u>ophthalmologist</u> at least once or twice a year to determine whether early problems are occurring.

"Chemotherapy" or "immune-suppressing" medications

In certain situations, when lupus causes serious or life-threatening problems, doctors may prescribe medications that depress the immune system. The following medications are sometimes called "chemotherapy agents" because they are also used to treat certain kinds of cancer.

- *Cyclophosphamide (Cytoxan)*

Use. <u>Cyclophosphamide</u> (<u>Cytoxan</u>) is used quite regularly for most forms of kidney inflammation. At the time of this writing, a treatment program using steroids plus cyclophosphamide intravenously (once a month for six months and then every three months thereafter for one or more years) is typically used. This regimen has been shown to prevent kidney failure more reliably than either steroids alone or steroids with other immune-suppressing medications.

Cyclophosphamide is also sometimes used for brain and neurological problems and blood vessel inflammation (vasculitis).

Side effects. This medication has a number of significant side effects, including stomach upset and nausea, hair loss or thinning, effects on blood and bone marrow cells, bladder inflammation and bleeding, susceptibility to infections, mouth sores, infertility and early menopause, and an increased chance of certain malignancies later in life.

High Blood Pressure and Lupus

Lupus itself does not cause high blood pressure, but if you have kidney inflammation, your blood pressure may be high. It is very important to control high blood pressure because it can lead to stroke, heart attack and heart failure, and it can further damage inflamed kidneys.

In addition, persons with serious lupus who require cortisone treatment can develop high blood pressure. The combination of lupus, cortisone and high blood pressure may increase the risk of heart attack and stroke. Therefore, regular blood pressure checks are important. Also, be sure to follow your doctor's recommendations for weight control, salt intake, exercise, stress management, and prescriptions for treating your blood pressure.

- *Azathioprine (Imuran)*

Use. Azathioprine (Imuran) is used in certain situations when lupus is severe. In some cases, doctors may use it to lower high doses of steroids.

Side effects. Azathioprine has a number of significant side effects, including nausea, liver inflammation, hair thinning, effects on blood and bone marrow cells, increased susceptibility to infections, infertility, and an increased risk of certain malignancies later in life.

- *Methotrexate (Rheumatrex)*

Use. Methotrexate is widely used in treating rheumatoid arthritis and a number of other conditions, and is gradually being used more in treating lupus. It may be especially helpful in treating arthritis, muscle inflammation, lung inflammation and severe skin disease. It may also permit a decrease in steroid dosage.

   Methotrexate is usually given once a week by mouth or injection. It doesn't depress the immune system as much as azathioprine or cyclophosphamide.

Side effects. It is usually well-tolerated, although it can cause skin rashes, mouth sores, stomach and intestinal upset, liver scarring, lung reactions (causing coughing and shortness of breath), fatigue, blood cell effects, and other side effects.

Blood vessel dilators

Use. These medications, also called vasodilators, improve blood flow when blanching of the fingers or toes (Raynaud's phenomenon) occurs. Blanching occurs when the blood vessels constrict and reduce blood supply. The medications open up, or dilate, the blood vessels.

   The most widely used medications for Raynaud's phenomenon are the "calcium channel blockers," such as diltiazem (Cardizem) and nifedipine (Procardia). They are available in once-a-day doses.

Side effects. Vasodilator medications may reduce blood pressure and can cause light-headedness, fainting, fluid retention, heart palpitations and nausea.

T here are many things that a person with lupus can do to help himself or herself. Keeping a record of the medications you take, preparing for upcoming exams, and planning wisely for work and pleasure can help you deal more effectively with the disease.

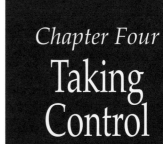

Medication Records

It is helpful to keep a record of the medications you take because they may be confusing and complicated. Your doctor will also be able to make sure you are taking the correct dose. A typical record might look something like the one below. The chart on page 38-39 has been prepared for your own use.

Recording Medications: A Sample

The sample record below illustrates one way that you can keep track of your medications, their dosages, and any side effects that may occur. The medications, if any, that your doctor prescribes for you will be based on your unique needs.

Medication	Dosage	Schedule	Possible side effects	Date started	Date stopped

Preparing for Your Next Exam

You may find that you can save time and receive better medical care if you are prepared to talk about what has happened since your last check-up. You can also prepare for your visit with the doctor by writing down all the questions you have had about your condition. It's easy to forget things that occurred and you didn't write down between doctor visits. The following charts show ways you might organize a personal "log" for this purpose.

Your Personal Record

1. Record any key symptoms and when they occurred.

Key symptom	When it started	When it stopped

2. Record all the medications you take. Include those your doctor prescribed, as well as any over-the-counter products you have taken. When you stop taking one, cross it off your list. Bring this list to your next office visit.

Medication	Dosage	Schedule	Possible side effects	Date started	Date stopped

3. Help to control your flares. After a flare has occurred, list any unusual medications you took. Think about what you did before the flare occurred.

Keeping such a record helps you and your doctor decide which, if any, products, medications, or activities you might avoid. You may need to keep these daily records for several months to uncover patterns that might predict a flare. Remember that most flares do not have any clear relationship to foods, activities, medications, or other environmental influences.

"Just before a danger sign or flare occurred…"

I used these medications: _____

_____

I participated in these activities: _____

_____

_____

I also remember I: _____

_____

4. List any questions you want to discuss with your doctor.

_____

_____

_____

_____

_____

_____

Preserving Energy

When planning your work and activity, always try to keep a little energy in reserve. Here are some tips to keep from becoming overtired.

• *Try to divide a tiring job* into smaller tasks — even if it means doing the job over several days.

• *Plan extra rest* when you know you're going to be working or playing hard.

• If you are going through a time of high stress, *take some emotional "quiet time"* for yourself each day.

• *Learn your limits.* Plan your work and activities so that you don't strain those limits.

• *Share with your doctor* any worries regarding the effect of your energy level on fulfilling job responsibilities.

• *If you need help in planning your work and activities,* your doctor might refer you to an occupational therapist or other professional. Your endurance can also be improved through regular exercise prescribed by your physician or physical therapist.

Career Choices

No career is absolutely off limits for someone with lupus. The most important thing to keep in mind when planning a career is the amount of control you will have over your work intensity and schedule. Lupus is a variable disease, and you should not expect to be able to perform at the same level every day.

If your job has flexible hours and allows you freedom to organize your daily tasks, you will be better able to deal with lupus flares. This arrangement works better than having to keep a rigid schedule.

Of course, some problems that people with lupus have may prevent them from doing certain things. For example, if you are short of breath, you probably shouldn't be involved in lots of stair climbing. Or if you have active arthritis, you probably should avoid lifting, repetitive hands or arms activities, and other motions that may aggravate the pain.

Travel Planning

Schedule your travel time wisely and pace yourself to avoid becoming overly tired. When planning a trip, remember to pack the following:

• your doctor's telephone number, your medical record number, and insurance information;

• the name and telephone number of a physician your doctor, friends, or relatives may recommend in the area where you are traveling;

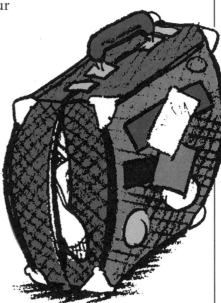

• medications, sunscreens and other items your doctor suggests (enough for the entire trip and extras for emergency delays);

• protective clothing; and

• some form of identification (in your wallet or on a bracelet, for example) with diagnoses, medications, allergies, doctor's name and emergency telephone numbers.

Many individuals with lupus live full lives. How do they do it? There isn't any "easy formula" for living well with a chronic disease such as lupus. However, those who successfully manage their disease share some traits:

They are active partners with their doctors, helping the doctors understand the symptoms and suffering that sometimes come from lupus.

Many people who have lupus give of themselves to their families, schools, careers, communities, and churches or synagogues. In doing so, they often receive more support than they would if they asked for it directly. And this helps keep lupus from being the center of their lives.

They learn about lupus and their personal limitations.

They recognize the need for lupus treatment and that such treatment can be complex. They agree to be responsible for their treatment and are careful to take medications properly.

They often tap into resources that can provide assistance, such as the Lupus Foundation of America, Inc., which has chapters in every state of the union. The Lupus Foundation offers support groups, educational programs and materials, newsletters, and other services. The Arthritis Foundation and Sjogren's Syndrome Association are other excellent resources.

They understand that they must nurture their psychological and spiritual health.

They realize that they can live well with lupus.

They learn to balance their lives. For example, they are not afraid to ask for help or understanding, but they do not overwhelm family and friends with their problems. They learn to balance rest and activity, work and leisure.

Alopecia Hair loss.

Anemia Low red blood cell count. If severe, can cause weakness, fainting, shortness of breath.

Antibodies Proteins made in the body that are normally sent into the blood to attack and neutralize bacteria, viruses, or other foreign substances and protect the body from them.

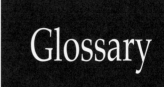

Anticardiolipin antibodies Special antibodies present in some people with lupus which increase the chance for blood clots to form in veins or arteries or for miscarriages to occur.

Anti-DNA antibodies A specific antibody test for lupus.

Antiphospholipid antibodies (APLAs) A group of autoantibodies seen in some people with lupus which increase the chance of blood clotting in veins and arteries and miscarriages. The three most common APLAs are anticardiolipin antibodies, lupus anticoagulant and the "false-positive test for syphilis."

Anti-Ro antibody See anti-SSA antibody.

Anti-Smith (anti-Sm) antibodies A specific autoantibody test for lupus.

Anti-SSA antibody Sometimes called anti-Ro antibody. Seen in some people with lupus or Sjogren's syndrome. Women with this antibody have a slight risk of having a child with congenital heart block (slow heart beat) or neonatal lupus. More severe rashes may occur in people who have this antibody.

Antigens Proteins or other substances that are usually foreign to the body. Antibodies form against antigens.

Arthritis Inflammation of joints.

Autoantibodies Antibodies directed against a person's own cells or tissues.

Autoimmune The characteristic of being physically sensitive to one's self. Autoimmune diseases are those in which the body's immune system reacts against its own cells.

Azathioprine (Imuran) A potent "chemotherapy" drug that depresses the immune system. Doctors use it to treat more severe lupus inflammation and to help lower steroid dose.

Chronic Lasting for many months or years.

Complement (C3, C4) A series of proteins (C3 and C4 are two of them) involved in system-wide inflammation. They are often decreased in people with active lupus or lupus nephritis.

Cyclophosphamide (Cytoxan) A potent "chemotherapy" drug that depresses the immune system and is used in kidney inflammation, neurologic problems, and vasculitis.

Cytoxan (cyclophosphamide) See Cyclophosphamide.

Dermatologist A doctor who specializes in diagnosing and treating skin diseases.

Discoid lupus A type of lupus affecting the skin only.

False-positive test for syphilis An antibody seen in some people with lupus. When present, it is associated with a higher risk of blood clotting in veins or arteries and miscarriages. This antibody does not mean the person had or has syphilis. Rather, the protein in the antibody cross-reacts with substances in the syphilis test. This cross-reaction makes the results a "false-positive" test for syphilis.

FANA test Stands for "fluorescent anti-nuclear antibody." Best screening blood test in lupus. It is positive in 95 to 98 percent of people with lupus.

Flare A time when lupus symptoms reappear or worsen; also called an "exacerbation."

Glomerulonephritis Inflammation of kidneys.

Hydroxychloroquine (Plaquenil) An antimalarial drug useful in controlling flares of lupus. It especially helps control inflammation of the skin, joints, and lungs.

Imuran (azathioprine) See Azathioprine.

Immune complexes Particles that form when antibodies attach to antigens. They may circulate in the bloodstream and deposit in organs and cause inflammation.

Immune system The body's protective system against germs, cancer cells, and foreign substances. It includes antibodies, white cells, lymphocytes, and other cells, proteins and chemicals.

Inflammation The body's reaction to foreign substances which enter it. Signs of inflammation are redness, pain, heat and swelling.

Internist A doctor who specializes in diseases that affect adults, usually involving "internal" organs such as the liver, kidneys, heart and lungs.

Leukopenia Low white blood cell count; if very low, the chances for developing infections increase.

Lupus anticoagulant Special antibody that may increase the risk for people to develop clots in veins or arteries or for miscarriages to develop.

Methotrexate A long-acting anti-inflammatory drug that is used in some inflammatory problems in lupus as well as other diseases.

Nephritis A short word for glomerulonephritis.

Nephrologist A physician who specializes in the diagnosis and treatment of kidney-related disease.

Neurologist A physician who specializes in the diagnosis of brain and nervous system diseases.

NSAIDs Stands for "non-steroidal anti-inflammatory drugs." These medications, including aspirin, reduce inflammation and can relieve pain. They do not contain steroids (cortisone-like medications).

Ophthalmologist A doctor who specializes in the diagnosis and treatment of diseases of the eyes.

Osteoporosis Thinning of bones. Many factors contribute to the development of osteoporsis, including age, calcium intake, menopause, and steroid treatment.

Pericarditis Inflammation of the sac surrounding the heart (pericardium).

Photosensitivity Being sensitive to sun or ultraviolet light. Many rashes seen in lupus are photosensitive.

Plaquenil (hydroxychloroquine) An antimalarial drug useful in controlling flares of lupus.

Pleurisy Pain in the chest that is aggravated by breathing deeply; it is usually caused by inflammation of the lining of the lungs (the pleura).

Raynaud's phenomenon Blanching of fingers or toes upon cold exposure due to constricting of blood vessels.

Remission A period when all the symptoms of lupus disappear.

Rheumatic Pertaining to aching of joints or muscles.

Rheumatologist A doctor who specializes in rheumatic diseases, such as lupus.

Sed rate Short for sedimentation rate, a blood test that reflects roughly the degree of inflammation in a person's body.

Sjogren's syndrome Inflammation of tear glands and saliva glands, leading to dry eyes and dry mouth. This occurs in some people with lupus or related illnesses such as rheumatoid arthritis, or by itself.

Steroids Powerful anti-inflammatory drugs. Doctors prescribe steroids most frequently when lupus inflammation is severe or resistant to other treatments. They are derivatives of cortisone, a hormone made naturally in the body by the adrenal glands. They have numerous side effects.

Systemic lupus erythematosus A chronic inflammatory disease affecting multiple organ systems.

Thrombocytopenia Low platelet count; if very low, may cause easy bleeding.

Vasodilators Medications that improve blood flow in constricted blood vessels; people with Raynaud's phenomenon frequently take these medicines.

About the Author

Eric S. Schned, MD, is the chair of the Rheumatology Department of the Park Nicollet Clinic, HealthSystem Minnesota, a large, integrated multispecialty group practice in Minneapolis, Minnesota. Dr. Schned's medical interests include lupus, rheumatoid arthritis and other connective tissue disorders, osteoporosis, osteoarthritis, fibromyalgia, and arthritis population health.

Dr. Schned is presently chair of the Board of Directors of the Minnesota Chapter of the Lupus Foundation of America, Inc. He has been a Board member since 1987 and also serves on the Medical Advisory Board of that organization. He is also chair of the Management Committee of the Park Nicollet Clinic and serves on the Board of Directors, HealthSystem Minnesota, and the Board of Directors, Institute for Research and Education, HealthSystem Minnesota.

Dr. Schned is board certified with both the American Board of Internal Medicine and the Subspecialty Board of Rheumatology, and he is a fellow of the American College of Physicians. He received his undergraduate degree from Yale University, New Haven, Connecticut, and his medical degree from Columbia University's College of Physicians & Surgeons, New York. Dr. Schned performed internship and residency duties at the New York Hospital-Cornell Medical Center and his fellowship in rheumatic diseases at the Hospital for Special Surgery, both in New York City. He served in the Indian Health Service from 1978 to 1979. He joined the Park Nicollet Clinic (then the St. Louis Park Medical Center) in 1981.